I0781380

Intermittent Fasting Diet Plan

Burn Fat, Stay Healthy and Live Longer!

Charles Kelso

Contents

Introduction to Intermittent Fasting

Fasting has a pretty long history behind it. Starting as early as 460 BC with Hippocrates of Cos, fasting was prescribed as a treatment for a number of symptoms. He wrote: "To eat when you are sick is to feed your illness."

Other Greek philosophers followed suit and were staunch supporters of fasting. This whole concept was born from observation of nature. When animals got sick, they did not eat, so fasting seemed to be nature's way of treating illness. Fasting is a universal instinct when dealing with sickness. Think about it. Last time you were sick, the last thing you wanted to do was eat.

Ancient Greeks also held a firm belief that fasting improved one's cognitive abilities. Consider how you feel when you overeat. Do you feel more energetic or sluggish? The problem is that most of us tend to overeat in today's world since food is so readily available. Overeating causes us to suffer from what's known as a food coma. Ancient Greeks noticed this long ago and came up with fasting as a solution.

There are also a lot of religions that practice ritual fasting. It's often associated with purification and cleansing of the body. It's believed to be extremely beneficial to the body. Buddhism actually practices a form of intermittent fasting. Often, they will only eat in the morning and then fast until the next day.

So we have established a little history behind fasting and why it's believed to be beneficial, but what does science have to say about it?

Why Choose Intermittent Fasting?
The reason is actually quite simple when you think about it. You should choose intermittent fasting because it will help you achieve your weight loss goals. Even though all calories are not equal, restricting them is the key to losing weight. When you fast, you make it a whole lot easier to restrict your calorie intake. It's probably the easiest dieting method to follow because it simplifies your day.

Rather than having to plan three to four meals every day, you will only need to plan a couple. This cuts your effort in half! It means that you have to make fewer decisions every day. You can also use these meals to

Introduction

enjoy larger portions, as long as you stay below your targeted daily calorie count.

Intermittent fasting will also save you money because you will be preparing fewer meals per day. More importantly, it saves you time. You only have to prepare two meals per day. That means you only need to do dishes twice per day. You only have to stop and eat twice per day.

Intermittent fasting also improves your insulin resistance and growth hormone secretion. These are two key elements to losing weight and building up muscle mass.

The human body is designed to fast for certain periods of time, so it is actually beneficial.

Part 1: What is Intermittent Fasting?

Chapter 1
The Science Behind Intermittent Fasting

Intermittent fasting is a pattern where individuals will cycle between periods of eating and fasting. Let's look at what science has to say about it.

Intermittent Fasting Shifts the Function of Cells
When you go without eating, there are several shifts in your body. Your body will initiate essential cellular repair functions, and your hormone levels will be changed in order to make fat stored in your body more accessible. Here are a few of the important changes:

- ➤ Insulin levels drop off significantly, which will cause your body to burn more fat.
- ➤ Your levels of human growth hormones can increase by a factor of five, leading to more fat burning and muscle gain.
- ➤ Your body can focus on cellular repair, rather than digesting food. This helps remove waste and cleans your system.
- ➤ There are a lot of beneficial changes to genes throughout the body that are related to protection against disease.

Most of the benefits of intermittent fasting are in relation to the changes in hormones and the way your cells act. The bottom line is that intermittent fasting initiates essential cellular repair processes and increased fat burning potential.

Intermittent Fasting for Weight Loss
Most people who try intermittent fasting are doing so to lose weight. I'm sure that's your goal if you're reading this book. We lose weight when we consume fewer calories than we burn. Since intermittent fasting causes us eat fewer meals, then we will be consuming fewer calories unless we overcompensate by overeating during those meals.

In addition to consuming fewer calories, intermittent fasting also enhances the function of your hormones, leading to the breakdown of fat. Contrary to the popular belief that fasting decreases your metabolic rate, this process actually boosts it by approximately ten percent. So we are essentially burning more calories.

So the criteria of burning more calories than we consume is being met.

Furthermore, one of the most dangerous fats is belly fat, and it's actually the first to go with intermediate fasting.

Intermittent Fasting's Effect on Insulin Resistance
One of the scary things about living in a world filled to the brim with processed foods and high sugary treats is the rapid jump in people suffering from type-2 diabetes. One of the scientific reasons behind intermittent fasting is that it has a positive effect on insulin resistance. Anything that reduces this resistance will help lower blood sugar levels and essentially protects from type-2 diabetes.

Intermittent fasting studies have shown that it has a big impact on the reduction of blood sugar in those who follow it.

The bottom line here is that intermittent fasting can protect from type-2 diabetes.

Intermittent Fasting Explained in Simple Terms

Intermittent fasting has become one of the world's go-to dieting trends. In short, it involves cycling through periods of fasting and eating. We have looked at the history and some of the science-based facts behind this lifestyle, so now let's take a closer look at some of the basics surrounding intermittent fasting.

So with intermittent fasting, you will cycle through eating and fasting, but there are no rules about what foods you should eat. What matters the most is when you eat. There are a lot of different fasting methods. They all split the day or week into two groups: fasting periods and eating periods.

Most people already fast when they are sleeping. Intermittent fasting just requires us to extend that period a little longer. You can accomplish this by skipping breakfast and eating your first meal at noon and your last meal at 8:00 pm. This method would have you fasting for 16 hours per day, restricting eating to an 8 hour window. This is known as the 16/8 intermittent fasting method.

Despite what most people tend to believe, it's not difficult to practice this type of fasting. It will actually boost your energy during this period once your body gets used to it. Hunger is usually not an issue either.

While you are allowed no food during the fasting cycle, you can drink water, coffee, or tea as long as it contains no calories.

You can also take supplements, as long as they contain no calories. The real key is that you allow your body to be cleansed during the fasting cycle.

Types of Intermittent Fasting

> **16/8 Method:** This method requires you to cycle through a 16 hour fasting period and an 8 hour eating period.

> **Eat-Stop-Eat Method:** This method requires you to cycle through at least one 24-hour period of fasting per week. However, two fasting days separated by at least a 48-hour period is recommended.

> **5/2 Method:** For two days out of the week, consume no more than 500 calories.

Note: *For beginners, I highly recommend the 16/8 method as it's the easiest of the three.*

Chapter 2
Intermittent Fasting Mythbusting!

I'm sure you have heard all of the noise surrounding healthy eating and improving your lifestyle. It's everywhere you look!

"Eating five or more meals per day is essential!"

"Eating throughout the day boosts your metabolism."

"Breakfast is the most important meal."

Let me ask you this: where did these beliefs begin? Why do you need to eat five or more meals per day? Why do you need to eat to boost your metabolism? Why is breakfast the most important meal?

I encourage you to research these statements yourself and look for evidence to support them. You're not going to find it! In fact, eating five or more times per day is what created one of the most obese generations the world has ever seen! Constantly eating forces the body to devote energy to digesting food rather than carrying out essential cellular repairs.

Here's a fact. In the '50s and '60s, people were eating three meals per day. When we doubled that in this generation, we saw the number of obese people grow. So evidence actually suggests the opposite of those beliefs. Humanity as a whole is not more overweight and less healthy than ever.

Let's look at some of the myths surrounding fasting in more detail.

Myth: Your Body Will Enter Starvation Mode

This might be the biggest lie to ever be associated with fasting. Fasting and starvation are not even close to being the same thing! Your body is not stupid. It knows the difference. Fasting is a choice that you are making consciously. You are in control of when it begins and when it ends.

An individual who is starving does not have a choice in the matter.

It's logical to conclude that your body is not going to go into starvation mode by not eating for a 24-hour period of time. This myth makes no sense.

Let's bust this myth back into the ground. When your body is fasting, your metabolic rate actually increases. It burns more calories, not less! Some studies have shown the metabolic rate of fasting individuals to jump up more than ten percent!

We actually see the opposite occur when individuals try to restrict calories. This is when the metabolic rate drops. Full on fasting does not produce this kind of drop.

Myth: Fasting Will Lead to Muscle Deterioration
First of all, it's important to understand that the body stores only two forms of energy—sugar and/or fat. That means the body can only use these two types of energy. Proteins are used to build muscle and are not used as a source of energy during fasting. The body will always use the easiest form of energy available, and the effort required for it to start breaking down protein is so great that it will only do it as a last resort.

Think about our history. When we were foragers, humans would go through long periods of time without eating. If their muscle were broken down, then they would have become weaker and slower. They were not weak or slow. Our very survival dictates that muscles should be a last resort for the body to use as fuel. They are not going to be negatively affected by fasting. Here's what actually happens:

> ➢ If your body goes 48 hours without food, it will start pulling from glycogen reserves. These are sugars that are easy to break down.
> ➢ After that, the body will start pulling from its fat reserves. Did you know that the average individual has at least 50,000 calories worth of fat stored? Do you know how long it would take the body to go through all of that fat?

Remember that the longest you will fast for is 24 hours, so this myth is completely unfounded.

Myth: Fasting Leads to Malnourishment

When you are in a fasting state, you are going to be at a calorie deficit—which is pretty much the entire point! But some people seem to believe that this can lead to malnourishment. In other words, we won't get the essential minerals and vitamins, leaving us weakened.

However, fasting for just 24 hours is not going to present a problem here. We are going to quickly replenish anything we lose when we eat. For fasts that last longer than 24 hours, then you can just take supplements to compensate.

This will not be an issue with intermittent fasting though.

The truth is that large food manufacturers put a lot of money into marketing to get you to believe that this will happen if you miss a meal.

Myth: After Fasting, the Food You Eat Will Turn into Fat

This is untrue. Here's what actually happens. When you break your fast, the body will look to restore its liver glycogen first. Since it can store up to 2,000 calories, it's going to start there. Plus, the liver is the easiest place for the body to access energy.

Since your body is always going to do what is most efficient, it will refill the easiest energy source first. Only when it has refilled those sources will it start using fat cells to store energy.

Myth: Breakfast is the Most Important Meal

We have heard this throughout our entire lives but does it really hold up to the facts? When we wake up in the morning, our body has been fasting the whole time we slept. It's okay to eat breakfast if you are hungry. But don't ever eat a meal just because people tell you that you're supposed to. Only eat when you are actually hungry.

Intermittent Fasting Mythbusting!

If morning is a time when you are fasting, then you should drink a tall glass of water. Most of the time, your hunger will go away because thirst can actually mask itself as hunger.

The most important meal of the day is not breakfast. The most important meal is when you break your fast. So if you are following the 16/8 method, then that meal will usually come around noon.

Part 2: How to Fast

Chapter 3
Different Intermittent Fasting Methods

Again, we have all heard that starting off with a healthy breakfast is the best possible way to lose weight. And if we want to lose even more weight, then we should eat five to six small meals per day. This is drilled into our heads from childhood into adulthood.

I'm here to tell you that there is more to the story. There is scientific evidence that shows skipping breakfast can actually improve the body's performance, physical health improvements, muscle retention, and even weight loss.

Those of you who are looking for a key to your weight loss struggles are in the right place because I'm about to drop some serious knowledge right into your proverbial laps. Let's start with a few of the common questions:

- ➢ Are intermittent fasting and keto dieting an amazing weight loss combination?
- ➢ What method should I use for fasting?
- ➢ Can I still fast if I work strange hours and exercise in the morning?

All three of those are amazing questions. Intermittent fasting can seem quite complicated when looking at it for the first time. The trick is to combine it with a well-balanced dieting plan. For instance, it will do you little good to fast for 16 hours per day if you are just going to eat a bunch of junk food during the eating cycle. You need to find an approach that works for your particular lifestyle and will help you meet your goals.

The biggest problem that beginners tend to run into is knowing how to make intermittent fasting fit into their life. Family, work, and your life in general can make it quite tricky to navigate. Fasting will only be a piece of the overall puzzle. You still have to make smart eating decisions.

Always keep in mind that intermittent fasting is not in itself a diet. It's a dieting pattern that you follow. You are making the conscious decision to skip certain meals on purpose. You'll be consuming all of your calories during a specific window.

With that in mind, there are several different methods of intermittent fasting to choose from.

Different Intermittent Fasting Methods

The 16/8 Method

This method requires you to fast for 16 hours per day and only consume calories within a specific 8 hour window. Most people will only eat from 12:00 pm until 8:00 pm when following this method, but you can adapt it to fit your lifestyle.

This is the absolute best method for beginners, so I encourage you to start here. It's actually my preferred method for long-term success.

You will basically skip breakfast and one other meal every day. Here are some examples:

- ➢ Your eating cycle is from <u>8:00 am until 4:00 pm</u>. After that, you will fast until the next morning.
- ➢ Your eating cycle is from <u>12:00 pm until 8:00 pm</u>. After that, you will fast until the next morning.
- ➢ Your eating cycle is from <u>3:00 am until 11:00 pm</u>. After that, you will fast until the next morning.
- ➢ Your eating cycle is from <u>7:00 pm until 3:00 am</u>. After that, you will fast until the next morning.

24 Hour Method

This method requires you to fast in a 24 hour window. For instance, if you finish eating at 6:00 pm, then you will not consume any calories until 6:00 pm the following day. You will repeat this once or twice per week.

This method can be quite powerful, but it is very difficult to maintain over the long term. This is the reason why I do not recommend it for beginners.

Those are the two most common intermittent fasting methods, so we're going to focus on them throughout this book. It's also worth noting that there are a lot of variations to those methods. Some people choose to eat in four hour windows, or even six hour windows. But I would say that you stick with the 16/8 method to make things easier on yourself.

By cutting out an entire meal or two each day, you are making it much easier on yourself to keep your daily calorie intake at a deficit, but that doesn't mean that you can just overeat during that window. It's important that you always remember that not all calories are the same. Plus, the timing of meals can also influence how the body reacts.

Intermittent fasting helps you lose weight because it forces your body to act differently. When you consume a meal, the body must devote energy to digesting and processing it. So individuals who are eating five to six meals per day are actually forcing their body to devote its resources to processing food rather than regenerating cells and other important tasks.

When you eat a meal, you are providing the body with easily available energy that it can burn, so it's going to choose that over burning its reserves.

However, in a fasted state, the body does not have recently consumed food so it is forced to break down fat cells as a source of energy. This is perfectly normal and is how the body is designed to operate.

Anytime you can burn fat, it's a win!

The same is true when you exercise while in a fasting state. Your body will be forced to get energy from the only source available. You guessed it! That energy is in your fat cells.

This works because the human body is biologically designed to react to the energy from food consumption by producing insulin. The more sensitive it is to insulin, the more efficiently the body will convert food into energy—and it's more sensitive to insulin after a period of fasting. This insulin sensitivity will cause you to lose weight and produce muscles.

Then to add on to that benefit, when you sleep your glycogen is depleted. More importantly, it's depleted during a workout too! This leads to an increase in insulin sensitivity.

<u>Meals following a workout are stored in a more efficient manner.</u>

When that happens, anything you consume will either be stored as glycogen in your muscles or burned immediately to help your body recover.

When you compare this to a standard day with no fasting, then the food and carbs you eat are much more likely to get stored as fat.

But that's not all. The production of growth hormones is increased when you are fasting, so when you combine this with the decrease in insulin production, you are essentially transforming your body into a fat burning, muscle growing machine!

To put this in simpler terms, intermittent fasting trains your body to use the fuel it gets in a more efficient manner. Your body will learn to burn fat for energy when you deprive it of new calories.

Now let's move onto a common question. Why do so many health books recommend we eat six small meals every day?

1. Every time you consume a meal, your body has to burn extra calories to process the food. But the problem is that it doesn't matter whether you consume 1,500 calories throughout the day or all at once, your body burns the same amount of calories to process it.

2. By eating smaller meals, you are less likely to overeat. This one actually does hold some merit, but the key to changing habits is to develop better ones to replace them. There is also an argument to be made that by eating smaller meals, you will never really be full, so you risk cheating anyway.

Chapter 4
How to Begin Your Intermittent Fasting Journey

One of the first steps that you will have to take on this journey is to set some initial goals. These goals should be simple and involve developing better habits. Most people will find motivation by defining their "why." Why do you want to start intermittent fasting?

We will also look at a few of the pitfalls that many people fall prey to so that you can avoid them. Without further ado, let's get started!

Intermittent Fasting Goals

One of the first things that we're trying to accomplish with intermittent fasting is to increase lipolysis. This will increase the fat burning potential of your body. We get most of the benefits from fasting from the last meal we eat before entering our fasting cycle. A lot of stuff will happen during that 16 hour window, starting with an increase in lipolysis.

Then the next goal is to boost cellular autophagy. This is the process where our body recycles proteins.

We will also force our body to produce HGH so that we are more sensitive to insulin. Fat burning and insulin sensitivity are directly linked to weight loss. When insulin is high, our body does not burn a lot of fat. However, when it's low, our body will burn a bunch of fat. So the goal is to become less sensitive to it so that our body doesn't have to raise the level of insulin it produces.

Avoid the Mistakes

As mentioned throughout this book, we're going to start with the 16/8 method, meaning that our fasting cycle will last for 16 hours. You can reduce or increase this timeframe if you want, but I highly recommend that beginners start with the 16 hour window. So now that those basics are out of the way, let's look at some of the most common mistakes that many beginners make when starting this journey.

Mistake #1: Not Consuming Enough Fat

Fat is an important part of fasting because it helps your body sustain its blood sugar level, essentially preventing reactive hypoglycemia. This condition is not good for your hormones. This is why healthy fats are really good, contrary to what so many people say. When you are fasting, you are not eating—and when you're not eating, you're not producing insulin.

Insulin is produced when we consume carbohydrates for the most part, although protein can also force us to produce it. However, it's rarely produced from fat. Fat by itself is not unhealthy. It's when you add all of those carbs to it that it becomes detrimental. My point is to make sure you are eating enough fat.

Mistake #2: Not Consuming Enough Calories
You should always start by calculating your daily calorie needs based on your overall goals. Then you must make sure that you get that amount of calories in that window. So many people will not eat enough during their window and suffer from it. They will usually get extremely hungry during their fast.

Remember that you are eating fewer meals, so you will need to eat more during each meal to make up the calorie difference.

Mistake #3: Experiencing Hormonal Issues
If you suffer from thyroid, blood sugar, adrenal, or hormonal issues, then cutting meals out of your day might not be a good idea because you are already stressed out. Not having those meals can lead to further levels of stress. The last thing you want to do is stress the body. That's another reason why the previous

mistake is so huge. Not getting enough calories is also a stressor.

My advice here is to get healthy before you attempt fasting. There are a lot of options at your disposal depending on your condition. Get your health issues dialed in, and then you can use intermittent fasting.

Getting Started in Five Easy Steps

Now we're going to take a closer look at how to get started on your intermittent fasting journey. Intermittent fasting is not complicated. It's actually quite a simple concept, but the execution can be a bit tricky. In short, you will be cramming all of your calories into an 8 hour window, which means you will be spending 16 hours fasting.

When starting on your journey, people are going to tell you that it's stupid and unhealthy. I heard it so many times that I almost believed it. Thankfully, I did not let those unfounded opinions deter me.

Let me make one thing clear before we begin. Intermittent fasting is not magic, so you cannot expect a miracle. Like any other change, it requires work and consistency. There are five fundamentals to making any dieting plan work, so we're going to apply those principles to intermittent fasting.

Step 1: Decide Which Method to Use
While there are several methods that you can choose from, we're going to focus on those surrounding the 16/8 method. The key with this step is to schedule your fasting time every day and then stick with it. So let me lay this out in a very simple way.

> Men should schedule 16 hour fasting windows. Make sure that your schedule is consistent.
> Women should reduce their fasting window to 14 hours. Make sure that your schedule is consistent.
> The fast should start immediately after eating your last meal. It should end with you eating your first meal.
> You should not consume any calories during your fast. This includes drinks that contain calories.

In most cases, the best meal to skip is going to be breakfast. For instance, you eat your last meal at 9:00 pm, then sleep from 11:00 pm until 7:00 am. You have already gone through 10 hours of your fasting window. So breakfast is going to be the only meal you really miss.

You can also decide whether or not you want to combine keto dieting with your intermittent fasting.

Use this time to go ahead and set your goals.

Do you want to lose weight?

Do you want to build muscle?

Whatever the case, write them down so that you have all of your goals documented.

Step 2: Calculate Your Calorie Needs
One of the most important parts of following through with intermittent fasting is to keep close track of your calorie intake. It's so easy to overeat during your eating windows. Always remember that in order to lose weight, you must stay at a calorie deficit.

Intermittent fasting is an amazing tool that makes it much easier to control your caloric intake. It makes the dieting experience more enjoyable, so it's much easier to achieve long-term success.

Another problem that so many people have is that they have trouble calculating their calorie goals. There are several ways that you can find this number but the best way is to just use an online calorie calculator. Here's a really good and simple calculator:

http://www.calculator.net

Once you have calculated your required calorie intake based on your goals, write it down. Documenting all of your goals will keep you on the right track.

Step 3: Calculate Macronutrients
You mostly hear macronutrients associated with the ketogenic diet but you should also use this information when following through with intermittent fasting. The fact is that all calories are not equal! It's important that you understand that simple, yet often overlooked fact.

Beginners might not necessarily have to worry about this, but I still recommend you go ahead and learn about macronutrients. That way, you can easily make changes to adapt your dieting strategy to your unique body. Here are some examples of how macronutrients make a difference:

> Consuming enough protein makes it easier for you to recover from workouts. You should consume most of your protein directly after a workout.

➢ Carbs can help your workout performance, but if you are combining keto dieting with intermittent fasting, then you will have to cut out carbs. You should always avoid carbs in the meal prior to entering your fasting window.

➢ Fat is essential to achieving your weight loss goals. I know that seems like a contradiction, but you should consume most of your fat just before entering your fasting window.

In order to achieve the best results, you should focus on more than just calories. These macros will depend on your overall goals. Here are two easy to use calculators.

Weight Loss: https://www.iifym.com/iifym-calculator/

Ketogenic Diet: https://www.ruled.me/keto-calculator/

Let's take a bit of a closer look at it all though. The following are basic macros for individuals who are not following the ketogenic diet.

Protein Intake

If your overall goal is to lose weight, then you should be consuming approximately one gram of protein per pound of your weight.

If you are obese, then you should drop that intake to one gram of protein per pound of lean body mass.

Fat Intake

> If your goal is to lose weight, then you should consume approximately 0.2 grams of fat per pound of body weight.

> To gain muscle, then you should consume approximately 0.3 grams of fat per pound of body weight.

Carb Intake

You should then comprise the rest of your calories with carbs. This is anywhere between 30 percent to 50 percent.

Macros for Ketogenic Dieting

Macros for keto dieting are actually easier to figure. Again, you can use a calculator to make this much easier. But here is a basic look:

Goal: Small Calorie Deficit (10%)

Fat: 73%

Protein: 21%

Carbs: 6%

Goal: Medium Calorie Deficit (24%)

Fat: 69%

Protein: 24%

Carbs: 7%

Goal: Large Calorie Deficit (36%)

Fat: 63%

Protein: 29%

Carbs: 8%

Of course, you never want to go above your calorie goals. You are simply spreading those calories among these macronutrients.

Step 4: Create a Meal Plan
All dieting plans tend to be thwarted by the most unexpected and simple issues—issues that are so stupidly simple that we never expect them to come up. For example, not having the right foods to meet out calorie intake for the day when we need them most. Or accidently miscalculating your calories—oops!

For this reason, I highly recommend you learn two important skills right now.

1. Learn to let it go. We all mess up, and it's fine. When you make a dieting mistake, learn from it, and move on. Do not let it completely thwart your plan.

2. Become a master meal planner!

Meal planning makes it so much more difficult for those simple things to mess you up. This is the simplest way to maximize your results!

Meal planning does not need to be boring or restrictive. You should plan in a way that gets you excited for your meals! Eat foods that you like and never get stressed about it. Remember, 90 percent compliance is better than no compliance at all. Here is a simple approach to meal planning.

1. Choose your recipes. There are some important things to keep in mind with intermittent fasting. You are going to be eating bigger meals than normal, since you're skipping one. You should also avoid carbs prior to entering your fasting window.

2. Choose meals that leave you with leftovers. This keeps you from having to cook as much and frees up time to do other things.

3. Make a shopping list. Never go shopping without a list because you will end up buying a bunch of junk. Another note is that when shopping, stick to the outer area as much as possible since that's where the fresh foods are located. Only travel the aisles when absolutely necessary.

Step 5: Create an Exercise Plan
First and foremost, this is entirely optional, but exercise can boost the results of any dieting plan, especially intermittent fasting! In fact, a lot of people who train heavily turn to intermittent fasting as a way to boost their results.

The best time to exercise is at the very end of your fasting cycle, when your insulin levels are low, and your body is relying solely on its reserves. When you train right after eating, the body has a higher insulin level, and it will use the energy from the meal to get the energy. This is okay, but not necessarily the most efficient method.

If you choose to work out right at the end of your fasting cycle, then follow up with a big post-workout meal. This will deliver the most optimal results!

The Bottom Line

There are so many people who are looking for shortcuts or magical methods of losing weight, and a lot of pill pushers tend to take advantage of these people. The problem is that the only way you are going to lose weight is if you consume fewer calories than you burn. This is the only fact that matters.

Intermittent fasting is not some quick fix. It's going to take effort on your part, but it is a powerful tool for accomplishing the only weight loss goal that matters, which is to remain at a calorie deficit.

Chapter 5
Intermittent Fasting for Health

Intermittent fasting is not limited to weight loss. It will actually improve your health in a significant way. Since you already know all of the basics surrounding intermittent fasting, we'll jump right into getting the most from this amazing practice.

Intermittent Fasting Improves Glucose Tolerance

Diabetics can use fasting to normalize their glucose and even improve their glucose variability. This is probably the most natural way of increasing your insulin sensitivity. You can expect to experience a significant difference in the way your body handles glucose once you have fasted for a few weeks.

Insulin resistance is usually the direct result of glucose being stored in tissues that are not built for fat storage. As the body burns through stored body fat, that accumulation will become smaller and improve your insulin resistance.

> ➤ To further increase insulin resistance, it's recommended that you consume most carbs right after you end your fast, preferably after a

workout. Of course, you can also combine intermittent fasting with the ketogenic diet for the best result.

Establishing a Routine

Strict eating times followed by a period of fasting can help your body develop a solid routine. The human body loves routines, so by giving it what it craves, it will function much more efficiently. Furthermore, you will be able to identify your own hunger cycles. This will help you develop better sleeping patterns, and you will even start scheduling your activities at more convenient times.

Establishing new routines is difficult at first, especially for those of us with a hectic schedule. But once you develop a consistent plan, you'll find that routines will actually improve your overall life.

> Set a strict schedule for your fasting cycle and your eating cycle. Stick to this schedule to the best of your ability.

Intermittent Fasting Boosts Your Immune System

This goes as far back as Ancient Greece where experts would recommend sick individuals to fast. Fasting boosts the production of white blood cells. Intermittent fasting gives your body 16 hours per day that it can focus on repairing damaged cells, rather than having to devote energy to processing food.

One of the myths surrounding fasting is that it weakens your immune system, but this is completely unfounded. Again, you're smarter than that. People tend to connect fasting to starvation, which are not even close to being the same thing. It takes quite a while before your body will enter starvation mode.

> Follow through with your fasting cycle, and make sure that you are getting all of the proper nutrients during your feasting window. You can also take daily vitamins to help.

Rejuvenate Your Skin

Those who suffer from acne have probably been told that the best way to regain control of it is through dieting. Processed foods and dairy are two big culprits of severe acne. Therefore, it should come as no surprise that intermittent fasting can also help you rejuvenate your skin.

Many skin conditions are caused by sensitivity to certain foods. Fasting can also benefit your hair and nails.

> After fasting, introduce different foods, one at a time, and monitor any changes to your skin. This will allow you to pinpoint the foods that are causing the most problems.

Intermittent Fasting Reduces Oxidant Stress

Oxidative stress is brought on by an imbalance in the production of reactive oxygen. This can lead to a number of sicknesses and has even been shown to cause cancer. Free radicals are unstable molecules that react with your important molecules like DNA, damaging it.

Overall, weight reduction that occurs from intermittent fasting will lead to a reduction in the body's oxidative stress.

> Help your body fight off this type of stress by following through with your fasting schedule. If you are obese, then I strongly recommend that you combine ketosis with this so that you lose the most weight possible.

Improving Your Heart Health

This is a big one. When you lower your body fat percentage, you are going to experience a ton of healthy benefits all throughout your body, but none is more important that the health of your heart.

Intermittent fasting will lead to a natural reduction in cholesterol levels. Plus, you will have some strain off of your kidneys as you lower your body's fat index. All of these factors will lead to a healthier heart.

> ➢ Try choosing heart healthy foods when possible to amplify this effect.

Boosts Healing and Recovery

Again, this idea goes all of the way back to Ancient Greece. Fasting will help boost your healing and recovery time from injuries. Exercise therapy at the end of your fasting window, directly followed by a large meal will boost its efficiency. Recovery is made simpler through intermittent fasting.

The reason is because we have a high sensitivity to insulin at the end of the fast, so the body will operate much more efficiently. We build muscle much more easily during this time. The bottom line is that fasting assists the body in recovery.

Time your therapy and workouts until the very end of your fasting window.

Chapter 6
Intermittent Fasting for Muscle Gain

Intermittent fasting can also be used as an amazing tool for muscle gain. The first important thing that I want to point out is that if you are looking to use intermittent fasting for muscle gain, then you should stick to the 16/8 method. Twenty-four-hour fasting cycles are not efficient if your goal is muscle gain. Sixteen-hour fasting cycles seem to work best for gaining muscle.

There are two main reasons why fasting helps our bodies produce muscle. Fasting raises our insulin sensitivity and causes our bodies to produce HGH. Again, creating too long of a fasting window will not help with muscle gain. It works for weight loss because it inherently lowers your calorie intake.

Someone using fasting as a muscle building tool would schedule their time to look something like this:

> **8:00 pm–12:00 pm:** Fasting Cycle
> **12:00 pm:** Exercise followed by a large meal
> **12:00 pm–8:00 pm:** Eating cycle
> **10:00 pm–7:00 am:** Sleep

Here is a quick look at the best approach to intermittent fasting for muscle gain.

1. Schedule Your Fasting Window

Your fasting window will be 16 hours, so let's go ahead and schedule that right now. Some people find need to slightly adjust this to fit their lifestyle, but 16 hours is the general goal you should shoot for. Laying out your plan is always the first step to any new endeavor.

It doesn't matter what time you schedule as long as it's a 16 hour period every day. The time should be consistent to allow your body to get into the routine.

2. Calculate Macros and Spread Them Over the Course of All Meals

Macros are usually the most confusing part of dieting for beginners, but there are online calculators that can help you. Once you have determined your macros, you should spread them out over the course of your meals. There are no rules here that are set in stone, but I do have a few recommendations.

- ➢ Eat most of your carbs during the first meal, immediately following your workout.
- ➢ Eat a meal high in fat and low in carbs as your last meal, just before your fasting cycle begins.

Again, those are not necessarily written in stone, but it's the most efficient way to lay out your meals.

3. Choose Your Workouts

Of course, if you want to build muscle then you will need to focus your workouts around strength-training exercises. Cardio and weightlifting are probably the two main ones you'll want to focus on. Remember that the efficiency of working out will peak at the end of your fasting cycle. The longer you practice intermittent fasting, the more efficient your body will become at utilizing other sources of energy to build muscle.

Also, it's worth noting that if you happen to rely on a carb-heavy workout diet right now, then you need to be careful when trying to combine high intensity exercises with intermittent fasting. Initially, you might run out of fuel since your body is used to being supplied with constant carbs. When you switch over the intermittent fasting, you might run out of glycogen reserves. Since your body is not used to using fat as a source of energy, you'll start feeling lightheaded and sluggish. It takes several days for your body to adapt.

4. Listen to Your Body

Finally, when you are fasting it is extremely important that you listen to your body. One of the biggest risks of intermittent fasting is low blood sugar, especially in the beginning. I do not recommend those of you who are new to fasting to take part in high intensity training. Start with low intensity workouts and then build your way up.

If you start to feel faint or lightheaded during your workout, then you should stop for the day. Bad feelings are your body's way of communicating problems to you, so you need to listen to it.

Key Takeaway

Most people simply dismiss intermittent fasting as a muscle building tool because of all the myths that have been drilled into their heads. However, it's actually one of the most powerful ways to build muscle. You just have to take certain steps to ensure that your body is given all of the nutrients that it needs.

Consider the fact that intermittent fasting is also one of the best ways to lose fat and you will see that it can be a life changing endeavor.

Chapter 7
Intermittent Fasting for Weight Loss

Again, you're probably hearing a little voice in your head screaming, "I need to eat six meals per day to lose weight. Skipping meals will cause me to gain weight!"

And again, I am going to reply with an astounding, "NO!"

There is not one piece of evidence anywhere that supports this belief. It's simply a myth that is the result of extremely effective marketing and poorly correlated studies done many decades ago!

With that said, there are numerous studies that prove fasting is a powerful weight loss tool. My point is that intermittent fasting does make weight loss much easier to achieve. Contrary to common belief, it does not slow your metabolism. It actually boosts it. In fact, let's start there.

Boosting Your Metabolism with Intermittent Fasting
The boost you get from fasting is anywhere from five percent to ten percent, which is actually pretty amazing. Another benefit is that fasting tends to get your body to

focus on getting rid of the dangerous fat around the waist and belly.

Intermittent fasting makes it much easier to keep your metabolism burning. All you have to do is plan your meals correctly in comparison to your fasting window. Always consume carbs at the end of the fast while consuming a lot of fat before you begin your fasting cycle.

Add exercise just before your first meal, and you will see an even bigger boost in metabolism.

Effects on Key Hormones That Lead to Weight Loss
One of the most effective weight loss effects that intermittent fasting has is that it optimizes the hormonal response of your body. One example is that it improves your insulin sensitivity, which is the primary hormone that the body releases when eating.

This is why working out right after a fast has such a powerful effect. You're pushing your body during a time when your insulin sensitivity is at its highest. The lower your insulin levels, the more weight you will lose. Intermittent fasting will naturally lower your insulin levels.

➢ To maximize this, be sure to exercise at the very end of your fasting cycle, followed up by a large meal.

Human growth hormone (HGH) is another powerful hormone that helps you lose weight and build muscle tissue. Fasting raises your HGH levels by a factor of 20, which provides you with phenomenal fat burning potential.

➢ To maximize this, consume most of your fats at the end of your fasting cycle.

Leptin is one of the primary hormones that tells you to stop eating and gives you the energy to exercise. Most people suffer from extremely low levels of this hormone, but fasting can actually normalize it. The bottom line is that you will have more energy and feel hungry far less often.

➢ Make sure you are eating all of your calories during the specified window. One common problem is that people starting out will not get all of their calories in.

Using Intermittent Fasting to Keep Lean Muscle

Maintaining your lean muscle tissue is an important step to losing weight. The more lean muscle tissue you have, the more calories your body burns at idle.

Lean muscle is amazing!

Intermittent fasting has been shown to be a much more effective method of maintaining lean muscle tissue than the standard calorie restriction diet.

> ➢ Just follow through with your fasting windows consistently, and your body will protect your lean muscle tissue.

Understand Why We Snack

Did you know that we snack mostly because we are bored and not because we're hungry? This a very important fact to keep in mind because it will completely change your life when you it hits you. While fasting, you're going to catch yourself getting up from your favorite chair and walking to the fridge without even thinking about it.

Everyone does this, but not everyone is conscious of it.

Our subconscious mind basically just wants us to do something, anything other than be bored. So you will find yourself being more productive while fasting once your brain understands that food is not an option.

> Avoid actual hunger cravings by eating a large meal just before you enter your fasting cycle. You should also try to work your fasting cycle around the times when you need to be the most productive.

Keeping Track of Your Calories is Important

Calories are always going to matter, so don't let some marketer try to convince you that there is some magic pill that will make calories irrelevant. You're smarter that that!

You must eat enough calories during your eight hour feasting window, but just make sure you don't gorge yourself on junk food. You will need to be aware of this danger at first because you are used to eating several meals through the day. This change can be a bit difficult for a few days, but once your body adapts, you'll be thankful that you stuck with it.

> Keep a food journal to track everything that you eat, along with the time you ate it. Your biggest meals should come directly before and after your fasting cycle.

Chapter 8
Intermittent Fasting for Women

One of the common questions about intermittent fasting is this: Does it have a different effect on women?

The answer is yes. Some women respond well to it while others report a slew of problems that arise. Like always, let's look at the science behind it, rather than just believing what people say.

Many healthcare professionals believe that fasting can improve a woman's health and is a safe medical intervention. But the impact of fasting on women does seem to be different than it is for men. We are all unique individuals, and our bodies are always going to be affected differently.

There are a number of circumstances when a woman should not attempt intermittent fasting. Furthermore, there is evidence that suggests that it's not as effective of a weight loss tool for women. That doesn't mean that women cannot gain the benefits of intermittent fasting. It just means that you'll have to pay attention to other areas as well.

- ➢ Focus on the quality of food you are consuming.
- ➢ Keep a close eye on your calorie intake.
- ➢ Exercise regularly.
- ➢ Get plenty of sleep.
- ➢ Drink enough water.
- ➢ Track your results!

Never attempt intermittent fasting if you fall under one of these categories:

- ➢ You are pregnant.
- ➢ You have a history of eating disorder.
- ➢ You suffer from chronic stress.
- ➢ You suffer from insomnia.

I am not saying any of this to scare women away from intermittent fasting. I just want your expectations to be clear going in.

Chapter 9
Tips for Continued Success

Intermittent Fasting Does Have a Couple of Drawbacks

There are not very many drawbacks to intermittent fasting. The main concerns seem to stem from what people believe rather than what actually happens. For instance, some people go into this with the idea that they are going to have less energy and feel hungry all of the time. They worry that they will be miserable because they are too hungry. But I like to look at facts, rather than just following whatever beliefs have become the popular opinion. In my experience, here are some of the drawbacks to intermittent fasting that you can expect.

The initial transition will jolt your system, but this is true of any lifestyle change. When you go from eating all of the time to fasting for most of the day, your system has to adjust to the changes. But your body will quickly adapt.

Some individuals also experience grouchiness when they skip breakfast. This is likely the result of breaking away from your past eating habits. If you are used to eating every three to four hours, then your body will get hungry until it adapts. This only takes a couple of days though.

Once it has been retrained to not expect food every three to four hours, then these side effects become less of an issue. In fact, you will start to feel more energized during your fasting cycle because your body is able to devote energy to other resources.

Intermittent Fasting is Not a Quick Fix!

It's extremely important that you do not go into this with the idea that intermittent fasting is going to just magically make you lose weight. You are not going to be able to fast, then eat 3,500 calories of junk food and lose weight. It's just not going to happen! This isn't magic—it's a dieting plan that is designed to promote a lower calorie intake.

If you tend to have an addictive personality when it comes to food, then you probably struggle with portion control. You need to track your calorie intake, and make sure that you are not overeating. If you consume more calories than you burn, you are going to gain weight.

Important Note: Intermittent fasting is more complicated for individuals who have issues with blood sugar regulation, suffer from diabetes, or are hypoglycemic. Individuals who fall into one of those groups should never try a new diet without consulting their doctor.

Muscle Gain and Intermittent Fasting

Contrary to the people who love to believe in myths, you can gain muscle while fasting. In fact, intermittent fasting actually makes it easier to build muscle mass. Let's use John as an example to see how workouts and intermittent fasting can be used in unison.

John would not lower his daily calorie intake, but rather than eating throughout the day, he would condense it into an eight hour window. The schedule would look something like this:

- **12:00 pm:** Intense strength training workout while still in a fasted state.
- **1:00 pm:** Consume approximately half of the daily calories for the day immediately after the workout.
- **8:00 pm:** Eat another meal, consuming the remainder of the daily calorie allowance.
- **9:00 pm-1:00 pm:** Fasting cycle.

This method is one of the greatest muscle building techniques on the planet! It's so much better than the standard techniques that are typically used. These techniques require an individual to overeat to build muscle before cutting their calories to lose weight. It's known as "bulk and cut."

Intermittent fasting is better than this bulk and cut technique for a number of reasons:

> Bulk and cut leads to some major weight shifts. An individual will put on 25 pounds and then cut off 20 pounds just to gain 5 pounds of muscle. Your body will get thrown out of whack. Intermittent fasting does not do this.
> Since you consume less food with intermittent fasting, you will be spending less money.
> It only takes small adjustments to stay within your goals.

So what can you do if you are working at noon and can't get in a workout? Believe it or not, this is a common question.

The 16/8 method can be adapted to any schedule. You can schedule it however you want as long as you are fasting for 16 hours straight every day.

Do not overthink it! If you have to train later in the afternoon or evening, then simply adapt your fasting schedule so that your fasting cycle ends just before your workout.

If you have to work out later in the day, but you break your fasting cycle at lunch, then you can modify your plan by making lunch a smaller meal that is high in fats and protein. Time carbs and big meals for after your workout.

There are a lot of ways to adapt intermittent fasting to fit any lifestyle. It's highly adaptable.

Intermittent Fasting and Keto Go Hand-in-Hand

Let's start by reviewing exactly what the keto diet is for those of you who might not know. In a nutshell, individuals following the keto diet consume only fat and protein. They are training their body to run efficiently by burning fat by eliminating carbs. This is a process known as ketosis.

There are actually two ways that you can enter ketosis:

➢ Eating foods that are high in fat and low in carbs.
➢ Fasting

The bottom line is that keto dieting and intermittent fasting are one of the most amazing fat burning combinations in existence!

When mixing keto with intermittent fasting, the body will enter the fasting state with no readily available sources of glucose. Therefore, the body will begin breaking down your fat into ketones. Fasting itself can also trigger ketosis, so your transition will likely be quicker when combining the two methods.

I personally believe that the sheer simplicity of fasting might be its greatest appeal. It shortens the window for making bad decisions. Add this to the simplicity of the ketogenic diet, and you have a lifestyle that is very easy to transition into.

On their own, both ketogenic dieting and intermittent fasting can be life-changing, but when you combine them, the opportunities are just off the charts. With that said, keto by itself is challenging. The concept is simple, but there are just so many opportunities to eat the wrong foods and get kicked out of ketosis. When you mix in fasting, then you eliminate some opportunities of messing up.

Tips for Continued Success

You need to decide what works best for you. We are all different, so what works best for me might not do the same for you.

Furthermore, you are not going to become keto-adaptive through intermittent fasting alone since your body will probably have enough glycogen stored. If you want to enter ketosis through fasting, then you would have to spend at least 24 hours in a fasting state. I personally find that it's much easier to stick to the 16/8 method and restrict carbs if you want to enter ketosis.

I encourage you to try different strategies to find out what works best for you. Just keep in mind that intermittent fasting is probably one of the only scenarios where you are almost always guaranteed to lose weight, as long as you track your calorie intake during the non-fasting cycle.

- You can use intermittent fasting to lose weight without the ketogenic diet.
- You can use the ketogenic diet to lose weight without intermittent fasting.
- You can combine the two, and lose more weight.

All options work. It just depends on your overall goals.

Fasting Tips

So by this point, we know just how powerful intermittent fasting can be to help you achieve your weight-loss goals. So now let's look at a few tips that should keep you on the right track.

<u>Don't overthink things.</u> It's human tendency to worry about new things until we adapt to them. Don't worry about whether eating an apple during your fasting cycle will ruin everything. If you do, then learn from the experience and move on. One slipup will not ruin your plan. The body is highly adaptable, so it will learn.

If you decide to eat breakfast one day and not the next, then that's okay for most people unless you're going for optimal athletic performance. Otherwise, stop overthinking, and don't let yourself stress over it. No one is perfect, and those who try to be are doomed to failure.

<u>Consider taking a walk in the morning while still fasting.</u> Taking a daily walk can be extremely helpful in helping you reduce your body fat. Plus, it will help clear your mind and prepare for the day ahead. Cardio exercises have a tendency to boost your metabolism too, giving

you more energy throughout the day. Morning walks are a good idea, regardless of what kind of dieting plan you are on.

Pay attention to your body, especially during workouts. If you listen to your body, then it will tell you what it needs. For instance, if you get light headed during a workout, then you probably need to consume more water. If your performance drops, then make sure you're consuming enough calories every day. If it gets severe during a workout, then pause it. You are allowed to ease into intermittent fasting.

Don't fall prey to peer pressure. Yes, that dreaded phrase still applies to adults. For instance, when you tell your colleagues or friends that you don't eat breakfast anymore, you can expect to get a lot of unsolicited opinions. Don't let them convince you that what you're doing is wrong. Breakfast's importance has been embedded into us throughout our entire lives, so people are going to believe that what you're doing is unhealthy. Just embrace it and move on. You'll prove them wrong by being healthier than ever!

Stay occupied. Rather than just sitting around pondering how hungry you are, get up and do something. You will struggle with this in the beginning, but your body adapts quickly. Here are a few ways to minimize your discomfort:

> Eat a large meal just before going into your fasting cycle.
> Consider that half of your fasting cycle will consist of sleep. It's tough to feel hungry while you're sleeping.
> Spend the remaining fasting cycle time after waking up doing something productive. You'll find that this is when you do the most work.

<u>Don't deprive yourself of life.</u> For instance, it's okay to drink zero calorie beverages during your fasting cycle. I don't care how restrictive some people say you "have to be," we're working toward developing better habits. We're not trying to completely restrict our lives! If you want some milk in your coffee, then add it. It's much better to live a lifetime of 90 percent compliance than it is to follow 100 percent compliance for only a month and stop because you were too restrictive.

If you want a diet soda sometimes, then drink it. In the beginning, do the minimum to keep yourself compliant. Once you have set some specific goals, then you might need to be stricter, but developing better habits is far more important for beginners.

<u>Always track your results.</u> This will depend on your goals. If you are trying to build muscle mass, then keep tabs on all of your strength training exercises to make sure you are actually getting stronger. If your goal is to lose body fat, then invest in some body fat calipers and keep a close eye on your composition. Always track your calorie consumption to make sure you are not going over your daily limit.

We all react differently to intermittent fasting so you will need to keep track of how it affects you. Listen, learn, and make adjustments as needed.

Do not expect miracles. Even though intermittent fasting will help you lose weight and boost your overall health, you cannot expect it to happen overnight. You must combine it with other healthy choices for it to work.

Putting it All Together

Intermittent fasting has a lot of positive benefits for your body but all of us are going to have different results. That's why I have pushed the fact that you must track your results all through this book. That's the only way to adapt it to fit your unique lifestyle. So let's put it all together now.

First and foremost, there is no "one size fits all" method for intermittent fasting. Let's recap the different methods that you have to choose from:

16/8 Method: You will fast for 16 hours and then consume your calories in a predetermined 8 hour window.

Fast for One to Two Days per Week: Eat normally for five to six days per week and then fast for one to two days. For instance, eat normally Monday and Tuesday and Thursday through Saturday, and fast on Wednesday and Sunday.

One thing that I have found quite common with those who try intermittent fasting is that they tend to struggle with knowing exactly when they should eat. They struggle with scheduling to the point that it stresses them out. So just relax and find a pattern that works best for you. Don't overthink it. The whole point is to start developing better habits. You can worry about the details   later.

Part 3: Nutrition

Chapter 10
Common Intermittent Fasting Mistakes

A lot of people have trouble with intermittent fasting because they fall prey to the same mistakes. Therefore, being aware of them right away is going to make this journey so much easier. So let's look at some of the most common intermittent fasting mistakes.

Eating Junk Food During the Window

So many people go into fasting with the idea that it's some kind of magic formula for solving their problems. Sure, it's a highly effective tool to take back control of your eating habits, but it is not going to help if you are eating a bunch of junk food. In fact, when following through with this plan, it's even more important than ever to make healthier choices. When you are fasting, the body breaks down damaged cells and uses them as a form of energy. This overall process will heal and cleanse the body. Your body becomes even more sensitive to what you eat, both good and bad. Furthermore, junk food will cause you to get hungry during your fasting cycle.

Calorie Restricting During the Eating Window

You should not restrict your calories during your eating window. If you need 1,800 calories per day, then you need to consume all 1,800 calories during this eight-hour period. The whole point of intermittent fasting it to get all of your calories in during that window. Your body will do amazing things if you simply do your job by providing it with the energy it needs.

Trying Too Much, Too Fast

This is an area where we all struggle when starting something new. Patience is the key to losing weight with intermittent fasting. You are not going to be able to pick up these habits overnight. You'll need to gradually work your way into fasting by setting small goals and working your way up to larger, more complicated ones. Your body must have time to adapt to the changes in your eating habits.

Trying to Be Perfect

One of the most important aspects of intermittent fasting is that it teaches you to truly listen to your body. In reality, our body only experiences real hunger every 16 hours. Your body should dictate when you eat, not a clock. The main focus is not to get everything perfect, but rather to develop self-awareness. Don't focus as much on the time period than you do on your own body.

Not Drinking Enough Water

When your body is in a fasted state, it will begin to break down damaged cells and detoxifies your entire body. It's essential that you flush those toxins out by drinking a lot of water. In fact, in the beginning you should make it a point to drink approximately 1.5 gallons of water per day. Then work your way down to around one gallon.

Chapter 11
Intermittent Fasting Fluids

Just like with any health and fitness program, there is no "one size fits all" method for intermittent fasting. There are a number of ways that you can adapt this strategy to accomplish your goals. So the next topic is going to be what you can drink during your fasting cycle.

In short, these liquids will not break a fast:

> ➢ Water
> ➢ Tea
> ➢ Black Coffee

Coffee

Let's start by taking a closer look at coffee. While coffee will not break a fast, there are certain things you can add to it that will break the fast. Black coffee is fine, but when you start adding sugar and cream, it can become a problem. Any beverage with sugar in it is going to break your fast.

You can add a high-quality source of fat to your coffee if needed. Some examples are coconut oil, butter, or MCT oil. Adding fat is actually really useful for those of you who are choosing to combine the ketogenic diet with intermittent fasting.

You can add fat and there is actually a limit on this. Never have more than one to two servings of coffee with added fat during a fast. This is what we call a "fat fast," where you are adding fat to your fast and achieving the same benefits. This really only works if you are mixing in the ketogenic diet though.

What About Artificial Sweeteners?
This is where things get a bit tricky. Most artificial sweeteners are marketed as having no calories, which means that they are not going to cause our insulin to spike. Fortunately, most artificial sweeteners are okay since they do not spike insulin, but they are still in a grey area. As a general rule of thumb, one or two artificially flavored beverages will not break your fast.

With that said, just don't overdo it. They are not exactly great for your overall health. I'm not saying that you have to eliminate them, but just limit them to one or two beverages per day.

Autophagy
This is one of the amazing benefits of intermittent fasting. When you can get into both a state of ketosis

while fasting, autophagy will occur. What happens is that the body recycles waste from the body and repairs oxidative stress.

It also has anti-aging properties and promotes the growth of muscles. There is a little concern from health professionals about black coffee and its effect on autophagy, but in my experience, this doesn't become an issue unless you overdo it.

What Other Liquids Are Allowed?
Let's start with one that a lot of people ask about—alcohol. As far as fasting goes, there are certain alcohols that are okay. Vodka is a prime example of one that will not break your fast. You could potentially get away with a glass of red wine if you're following the ketogenic diet, but you should avoid it during your fasting cycle.

It's just best to keep alcohol to a minimum since it can have adverse effects on your hormones, which is one area that you are trying to improve through fasting.

<u>**Key Takeaways**</u>

Intermittent Fasting Fluids

- Water, tea, and black coffee will not break your fast so you can drink them.
- You can add healthy fat to coffee if you drink it in moderation. No more than one to two servings per day.
- Artificial sweeteners are a grey area and should be consumed in moderation. No more than one to two servings per day.
- Sugar is not allowed and will break your fast.

Chapter 12
Best Foods to Eat with Intermittent Fasting

By this point, I have gone through many of the details associated with intermittent fasting, but here is a quick recap. Intermittent fasting is highly adaptable. There are dozens of ways that you can approach it. I have given you my personal recommendation, but that is not set in stone.

This section is going to focus on some of the different foods that you can consume while following this strategy.

Finding the Best Foods
There are really no food specifications with intermittent fasting. All you're doing is creating windows where you do not eat any food. The food restrictions only come into play when you are combining it with another diet, like ketogenic, for example. Naturally, if you are combining keto with intermittent fasting, then you would need to avoid foods that contain carbs.

You should also keep in mind that you should stay away from horribly unhealthy foods. Fasting will do little good if you are eating Big Macs when you're not fasting. Try to stay away from processed foods as much as possible.

To make things easier on you, I will discuss a few foods that can be included as part of a healthy eating lifestyle.

Avocado

Yes, avocados are high in calories, but they contain monounsaturated fat, which make them extremely filling. You can eat half an avocado for lunch and stay full for hours. If you are following the ketogenic diet, then avocados are one of the best foods because of their high healthy fat content.

Fish

A lot of diets highly encourage you to eat fish, and for good reason. Fish contains the healthiest fats and proteins. Fish is also considered one of the healthiest brain foods on the planet! So if you are limiting your calories every day, then you might as well get the most from what you do eat. Fish delivers the most bang for your buck!

Cruciferous Vegetables

Broccoli, brussels sprouts, and cauliflower are three of the most amazing veggies you can eat. They contain a ton of fiber and are usually allow on any dieting plan.

Those of you who understand keto dieting know that fiber does not count toward your net carbs. Furthermore, fiber will make you feel fuller for longer.

Potatoes

This is strictly for those of you who are not following the ketogenic diet. Potatoes are a satiating food, and alone, they are very healthy. It's only when we fry them or add a lot of unhealthy topping that they become a detriment. I recommend you reserve potatoes for the meal directly following your fasting cycle.

Beans and Legumes

Again, this is fair game for anyone who is not following the ketogenic diet. Why not throw some low calorie carbs into your meal plan? They provide energy and will keep you fuller for longer. Plus, they are high in fiber. Beans have also been shown in several studies to help with weight loss. Just like potatoes, I recommend you reserve beans and legumes for the meal directly following your fasting cycle.

Berries

Berries are loaded with vital nutrients. For instance, strawberries are an amazing source of vitamin C—more than 100 percent of your daily value in just one cup!

That's not even the healthiest part! Flavonoids like strawberries and blueberries have been shown to provide BMI increases in several studies. However, you will have to be careful with berries if you are following the ketogenic diet.

Eggs

Eggs are one of the cornerstone foods of the ketogenic diet. They can be cooked in minutes and contain both protein and fat, both of which are important to building muscle. Strength trainers eat eggs religiously due to their powerful effects. You can consume eggs right before you enter your fasting cycle and stay full for quite a while.

Nuts

Nuts are higher in calories than most snacks, but they also contain healthy fats. These can be a really good way to round off your calories while following through with intermittent fasting. They make for a great snack in-between meals. Just be careful with how many nuts you consume because they are loaded in calories.

Whole Grains

Once more, if you are on the ketogenic diet then whole grains are out of the question. But they do have a lot of healthy properties, including that they are rich in both protein and fiber. A little bit of whole wheat goes a long way. Plus, whole grains have been shown to boost metabolism, another plus for those following intermittent fasting.

Chapter 13
Combining Ketogenic Dieting with Intermittent Fasting

Intermittent fasting and the ketogenic diet are both extremely popular weight loss methods that have grown in popularity over the past few years. Individually, they hold a lot of potential for weight loss, gaining lean muscle mass, and can even boost your energy levels. However, now we're going to take it a step further and combine these two powerful methods. Fasting while on the ketogenic diet will provide a significant boost to your results and provides amazing health benefits.

Let's start by going over some of the basics.

Fed State Versus Fasting State

Eating every few hours (like almost every other diet preaches) puts you into what we're going to call the "fed state." When you are in the fed state, your body is devoting most of its energy to digesting, absorbing, and storing nutrients from the food you have consumed. Most of us remain in this state all day except while sleeping. Your body does not focus on burning fat during the fed state.

The main reason why intermittent fasting works is because it puts the body into a fasted state. This state forces your body to burn fat and frees it up to perform essential cellular repair.

Why Combine Keto and Intermittent Fasting?
Let's look at a few of the benefits of combining these two powerful weight loss tools.

You Will Enter Ketosis Sooner
With the ketogenic diet, you are essentially fasting yourself from carbs and glucose. So, fasting for 16 hours per day will help you get into ketosis much faster because you are essentially expanding on the same concept. You are kick-starting your body into ketosis.

You will also find it much easier to fast for longer periods of time while you are in a state of ketosis since your body has already trained itself to use fat as a primary source of energy.

Accelerated Weight Loss
The keto diet is an amazing weight loss tool on its own. By removing carbs from your diet, you are training your body to burn fat rather than depend on glycogen. High fat diets are also much more saturated, and they will

make you feel full for longer. This keeps your hunger under control.

When you combine this with intermittent fasting, you will have an even shorter window for eating. This allows your body to use the food that it consumes as fuel without you feeling hungry or deprived. In short, it's so much easier to remain at a calorie deficit, which is the only way you lose weight.

Balancing Your Blood Sugar
Both the ketogenic diet and intermittent fasting will improve your insulin sensitivity. This lowers your blood sugar levels, which is a crucial step to losing weight. These benefits combine to stabilize blood sugar even faster than normal. This would be great for anyone suffering from type-2 diabetes.

When you stabilize your blood sugar levels, you also have a clearer mind and can focus better.

How to Combine Fasting with Ketogenic Dieting

As I have said several times throughout this book, there is no right or wrong way to do intermittent fasting. I highly recommend fasting in 16 hour windows, but it's not set in stone. I am going to show you my favorite method for combining fasting with the ketogenic diet, but remember that you might need to modify it slightly to fit your unique needs.

When fasting, listen closely to your body. It will tell you whether you need to reduce or expand that window.

If you experience low energy levels for at least a week, then you know that you need to modify the window.

If you find that you are extremely hungry throughout the fasting cycle, then you might need to shorten it and add an hour to it every week or two until you hit your target.

You should also make sure that you are getting in all of your daily calories during your eating window. A lot of people will simply not eat enough and then wonder why they feel awful during their fast. The goal with intermittent fasting is to get in all of your calories within a short window.

Combining ketogenic dieting with intermittent fasting works in the same way. You are trying to stuff all of your calories into a short window. The difference is that you are not introducing carbohydrates into your system.

Step 1: Find your Macros

Most dieting plans do not really require you to worry about macronutrients. I mean understanding them is a bonus, but it's not hugely important. However, when following the ketogenic diet, knowing your macros is essential–dare I say even more essential than counting calories?

Fortunately, there are a lot of calculators online that can help you determine your macros. You are going to have to keep track of this information. The problem is that a lot of people will lie about their body fat index, and they end up calculating macros that do not contain enough calories. With fasting, it's essential that you consume all of your daily calories.

A macro calculator will have you put in the following information:

- Weight and Body Fat Index
- BMR and TEF (calories you burn at idle)
- Your Daily Activity Level
- Daily Exercises
- Dieting Goals
- Protein Ratio (dependent on activity level)

The calculator will then spit out your macro. This will show you the percentage of calories you should be getting from fat, protein, and carbs.

Here's where things get a bit tricky. Eating all of those calories within an eight-hour window is not going to be easy for those of you who are just starting out. You will have to pay close attention to what you are consuming.

Starting a low carb diet changes us and our kitchen cabinets. No, we don't mean resurfacing or new hardware. Take an honest inventory, and make some changes for your new low carb diet.

Step 2: Create a Failproof Kitchen
Here, we're going to carb-proof the kitchen so that you do not fall prey to cravings and temptation. Most people go into a dieting plan, but they do not clean out their pantries. They count on willpower alone to get them through it. Let me be the first to tell you that willpower is not stronger than biology. You will not be able to overpower your biological craving of carbs through willpower alone. Eventually, you will lose, so clear out all of that temptation so that you don't have to fight this battle.

Get rid of all high carb foods. Be brutal! All of those processed cereals, rice, and candies must go. I encourage you to donate them to a local charity. You are allowed to keep processed foods that are low in carbs, but I recommend that you limit all processed food choices.

One issue that comes up quite often is when others in the household are not following a ketogenic diet. If a roommate or significant other is still using high carb foods, then create your own space in the kitchen. Separate all high carb food choices from your area of the kitchen.

When following the ketogenic diet, you will be eating more meats and produce that anything else, so it's important that you clear space in your fridge and equip yourself with a lot of storage containers.

For instance, barbecue sauce is forbidden on the ketogenic diet since it's loaded with sugar. You'll basically be replacing your customary foods with low-carb choices.

Some of those who are new to the ketogenic diet have a tough time giving up sweet treats and easy lunches. Here are some alternatives:

Low-Carb Bread: There are a lot of different types of low-carb bread. You can usually find them in the health section of the store. In my supermarket, there is a type of bread that costs $7 per loaf, but it contains no net carbs. It contains seven grams of fiber, which does not count towards the ketogenic diet.

Low-Carb Chocolate: You can also find low-carb chocolate to curb your sweet-tooth. It's available in the health section in most supermarkets. Furthermore, you can also eat small amounts of dark chocolate. Just pay close attention to the serving size.

Step 3: Your First Shopping Trip
Once you have gotten rid of the old, it's time to replace it with new, healthier options. You must have foods in the kitchen that support your low-carb lifestyle. The absolute worst situation is to be hungry without anything appropriate to eat. A low-carb lifestyle requires you to have certain items that you can quickly and easily whip up so that you are able to get in those calories

during the right windows. Here are some of the items that you should buy during your first shopping trip.

Beverages
Water is the absolute most important drink for all diets. You should always make sure you are drinking enough water every day. You can even flavor up some of your water with Splenda-flavored packets. Another really good beverage to support weight loss is coffee, as long as you are not adding sugar to it. Tea is another great choice. What makes all three of these beverages so amazing is that they are also all approved to drink during your fasting cycle.

Cheese
There are a lot of different types of cheeses available that you will find that it becomes the go-to snack for your low-carb lifestyle. Shredded cheese is perfect for adding essential fat to your meals. You can also combine it with meats to give you a satiating snack. It's one of the staples of the ketogenic diet.

- Cheddar cheese
- Mozzarella cheese
- Cream cheese
- Bleu cheese

- ➢ Parmesan cheese
- ➢ Cream spinach cheese

Keto-Friendly Vegetables

Broccoli and spinach should always be on-hand in the kitchen to add to your favorite recipes. Just remember that not all veggies are created equally. Some of them are not going to meet your low-carb needs. As a basic rule of thumb, stick with veggies that are above ground.

You can even use cucumber slices and cauliflower for snacking. Either eat them with a low carb salad dressing or steam them and top with cheese.

- ➢ Green peppers
- ➢ Onions
- ➢ Cauliflower
- ➢ Spinach
- ➢ Scallions

Fresh Meats (Protein)

Don't be afraid to explore different types of meat. Try new things and make sure that your kitchen doesn't get boring! Fish is an often overlooked meat that has amazing health benefits associated with it. You will just want to avoid certain deli meats and processed meats like hot dogs. If you are in doubt, just check the label.

➢ Ground beef

➢ Sausages

➢ Chicken Breast

➢ Ham (no-added sugar)

➢ Bacon

➢ Eggs (not necessarily a meat, but high in protein)

Fats

Fats are the foundation of the ketogenic diet, and you should consume a lot of these just before you begin a fasting cycle. You will want all of your recipes to be heavy in fat, so make sure that your kitchen is equipped with these fats.

➢ Heavy cream

➢ Olive oil

➢ Coconut oil

➢ Unsalted butter

➢ Sesame Oil

Putting it All Together

One of the important things about following through with intermittent fasting is cramming all calories into an eight-hour window. It's makes things a little more complicated, but I promise that the effort will be well worth it once you start to see that weight rapidly drop off.

Let's look at a typical day:

Breakfast
When you wake up, you will already be most of the way through your fasting cycle, so you can start your day off with a keto-proof coffee to help give you that boost to get you through the rest of the window. This involves you adding some kind of fat to the coffee, like coconut butter, for example. As mentioned earlier in the book, it will have a few calories, but it will not break your fast since it's all from fat. Just do not drink more than one cup.

Keto-proof gives your metabolism a jolt and will help give you the energy to tackle the morning. Plus, you are fueling your fat burning potential, which is what fasting does. That's why these calories are okay. They support everything that we're trying to accomplish with intermittent fasting.

Finally, make sure that you keep track of this morning coffee in your macros.

Lunch

This is where you will be breaking your fast, so if you are planning to exercise, the perfect time to do so is just before eating lunch. Follow it up with a large meal. I recommend that you try to get in at least forty percent of your daily calories here.

This large lunch is going to be used as energy immediately so it will give you a significant metabolic boost. You can also have a caffeinated drink now or another keto-proof coffee if you want. You're going to want to get as big of a metabolic jump as possible. Lunch should focus more on fat than protein.

Dinner

Your last meal before entering the fasting cycle should contain the bulk of your calories. It should possess cheese, fats, butter, and other oils. This is actually the trickiest part of this dieting plan because we have to make sure we get enough protein in our system to last through the fasting cycle.

Here, we're going to be focusing more on protein here, which goes against the grain a bit when dealing with the ketogenic diet. So it's important that you keep track of your daily macros so that you can make sure you're getting them right throughout the day.

The reason we need protein just before a fast is because it keeps us full for longer, and it helps maintain lean muscle mass.

You want a meat like chicken as your main course. Then add butter, cheese, sauces, and oils to give it a good dose of fat. You can even make a side salad to go with your meat to introduce more fat to the meal.

No Snacking While Fasting

Okay, so snacking is a grey area. You should try your best to stay away from snacking during your fasting period because it interrupts the process. However, you also have to listen to your body. If you feel lightheaded or dizzy, then you might need a small snack to carry you over.

The problem with snacking is that it leads to hunger. If you need to snack, then get a palm full of nuts. Just make sure that you don't repeat this behavior every day.

Chapter 14
Sample Meal Plan

Now we're going to take a look at a sample meal plan that I have put together to give you an idea of what you can expect when combining intermittent fasting with the ketogenic diet. Keep in mind that if you do not have a lot of time to cook during the week, then you can cook a week's worth of food, store it in freezer Tupperware, and then just microwave it when you get ready to eat.

Two important parts to this plan are that you get in all of your calories during the eating cycle and that your food has variety. Not adding variety to any diet will cause you to quickly get bored of it. When you get bored, you start looking in all of the wrong places for entertaining food choices.

There is no reason to follow this sample meal plan exactly as listed. You might find that you need fewer calories per day than what I am recommending. Plus, if you are drinking keto-proof coffee, then you are gaining a lot of calories there.

Day 1
Fasting Cycle: 7:00 am–12:00 pm

Workout: 12:00 pm–12:30 pm

Lunch: <u>Low Carb Pizza </u>(immediately following workout)

Dinner: <u>Keto Fried Chicken</u> (8:00 pm followed by fasting cycle.)

Fasting Cycle: 8:00 pm–7:00 am

Day 2
Fasting Cycle: 7:00 am–12:00 pm

Workout: 12:00 pm–12:30 pm

Lunch: <u>**Chorizo Cheddar Meatballs** </u>(immediately following workout)

Dinner: <u>Buffalo chicken with paprika mayo and butter-fried cabbage</u>

(8:00 pm followed by fasting cycle.)

Fasting Cycle: 8:00 pm–7:00 am

Day 3
Fasting Cycle: 7:00 am–12:00 pm

Sample Meal Plan

Workout: 12:00 pm–12:30 pm

Lunch: <u>Low Carb Pizza</u> (immediately following workout)

Dinner: <u>Keto Fried Chicken</u> (8:00 pm followed by fasting cycle.)

Fasting Cycle: 8:00 pm–7:00 am

Day 4

Fasting Cycle: 7:00 am–12:00 pm

Workout: 12:00 pm–12:30 pm

Lunch: <u>Chorizo Cheddar Meatballs</u> (immediately following workout)

Dinner: <u>Buffalo chicken with paprika mayo and butter-fried cabbage</u> (8:00 pm followed by fasting cycle.)

Fasting Cycle: 8:00 pm–7:00 am

Day 5

Fasting Cycle: 7:00 am–12:00 pm

Workout: 12:00 pm–12:30 pm

Lunch: Sweet and Sour Chicken (immediately following workout)

Dinner: Keto chicken fajita bowl (8:00 pm followed by fasting cycle.)

Fasting Cycle: 8:00 pm–7:00 am

Day 6

Fasting Cycle: 7:00 am–12:00 pm

Workout: 12:00 pm–12:30 pm

Lunch: Bacon Wrapped Chicken Cordon Bleu (immediately following workout)

Dinner: Bacon-wrapped keto burgers (8:00 pm followed by fasting cycle.)

Fasting Cycle: 8:00 pm–7:00 am

Day 7

Fasting Cycle: 7:00 am–12:00 pm

Sample Meal Plan

Workout: 12:00 pm–12:30 pm

Lunch: <u>Bacon Wrapped Chicken Cordon Bleu</u> (immediately following workout)

Dinner: <u>Eggceptional Sausage Keto Frittata</u> (8:00 pm followed by fasting cycle.)

Fasting Cycle: 8:00 pm–7:00 am

<u>Note:</u> If you are just starting out, then you can just follow through with the morning fast and wait a week or two to add in the nighttime one. Remember, you'll be sleeping most of that time anyway.

Week 2

For the purpose of making this as simple as possible, you can follow the same meal plan as the previous week. Or you can sub out foods you like for foods you don't like. We're trying to develop better habits at this point, not get everything perfect.

Again, you can wait another week to extend your fasting cycle if you want.

Weeks 3 and 4

This is when you will need to start getting more aggressive by following through with the entire 16-hour fasting cycle. Get in all of your calories during the eating window. You might also improve your results by halving your keto-proof coffee so that you can put those calories into nutrients. If you need more coffee, then drink it black. Here are some tips to keep in mind as you move forward:

> ➢ It's essential that you stick with the same routine every day. Let your body get used to it.
> ➢ Absolutely no snacking during the fasting cycle once your body has gotten used to it.
> ➢ Drink plenty of water! It's essential that you stay hydrated.
> ➢ You are allowed to eat desserts. Just be sure that they are keto friendly and that you keep your macros in mind.

Conclusion

Like I have said throughout this book, one of the first mindsets that you have to overcome is the false belief that fasting and starving are the same. They are not. Yet, we have been raised in a way that when we miss a meal, our mind falls back to that old adage, "I'm starving!"

We are trained to eat every meal, every day, as kids. We are taught that skipping a meal is unacceptable. But by now, you all know that is simply not true.

With that in mind, I recommend that those of you reading this book slowly develop better eating habits as you begin your intermittent fasting journey. Don't try to do it all at once. It's going to be extremely difficult to fast for 16 hours right away unless you already follow consistently healthy eating habits.

Here are some final tips to keep in mind:

➢ Most beverages should contain no calories. Water, unsweetened tea, and black coffee are all great choices.
➢ Most meals should contain a good source of protein.

> Most meals should contain at least one serving of vegetables.
> Most meals should include a healthy fat.
> You should consistently get between seven to nine hours of sleep every day.
> More carbs should be eaten just after your fasting cycle.
> More fats should be eaten just before your fasting cycle.
> You should keep a food journal for the best results.
> Exercise is a bonus but not a requirement. It will enhance your results. Think of it like extra credit work at school.

You can always spend a week tracking your food intake to see if you are following consistently healthy eating habits. Usually, if you are unsure then you are not being healthy.

Intermittent fasting is not some magic formula that's going to make up for poor eating choices, so you must develop better habits. If you are looking to create better habits, then you now have the tools to help you do just that.

About the Author

Charles Kelso is a professional health coach who shares his secrets in order to help others achieve their goals. He understands just how important it is to relay accurate information to his clients, rather than just following along with whatever is today's trend.

Charles has helped hundreds of people achieve phenomenal success using his highly successful strategies, many of which are found in this book. He hopes that it can will help you too!

One Last Thing… Did You Enjoy the Book?

If so, then let me know by leaving a review on Amazon! Reviews are the lifeblood of independent authors. I would appreciate even a few words from you!

If you did not like the book, then please tell me! Email me at lizard.publishing@gmail.com and let me know what you didn't like. Perhaps I can change it. In today's world, a book doesn't have to be stagnant. It should be improved with time and feedback from readers like you. You can impact this book, and I welcome your feedback. Help me make this book better for everyone!

Conclusion

Copyright 2017 by Charles Kelso - All rights reserved.

All Rights Reserved. No part of this publication or the information in it may be quoted from or reproduced in any form by means such as printing, scanning, photocopying or otherwise without prior written permission of the copyright holder.

Disclaimer and Terms of Use: Effort has been made to ensure that the information in this book is accurate and complete, however, the author and the publisher do not warrant the accuracy of the information, text and graphics contained within the book due to the rapidly changing nature of science, research, known and unknown facts and internet. The Author and the publisher do not hold any responsibility for errors, omissions or contrary interpretation of the subject matter herein. This book is presented solely for motivational and informational purposes only.

www.ingramcontent.com/pod-product-compliance
Lightning Source LLC
Chambersburg PA
CBHW031310250726
48656CB00005B/1722